# Angelic-Reiki Energy Healing™

# Course Work
# And Permission Forms

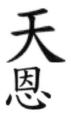

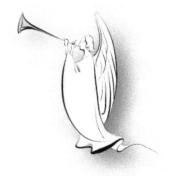

# By the Grace of God, Go I

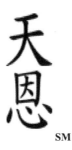
SM

The top symbol represents

**GOD**

Our Divine Creator

The other symbol represents

**GRACE**

May the Grace of God find favor in you.

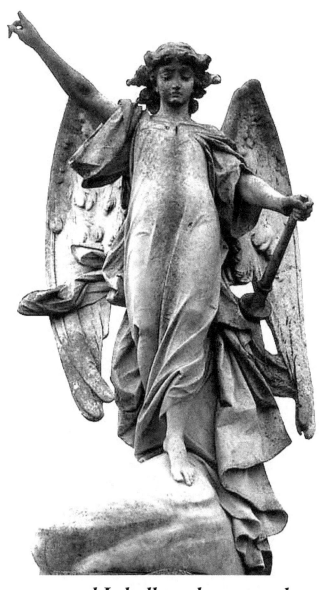

*. . . and I shall send you angels*
*to guard you, to guide you,*
*and to bless you*
*Indeed*

# ACKNOWLEDGEMENTS

This book, as all my books are dedicated to
My Guards and My Guides
The Powers That Be
With My Gratitude
Be Blessed
Indeed

Angelic-Reiki Energy Healing
Written By
Rev. Debbie Michaels
Subject to copyright ©

**Contact the author at…
AngelsGather88@hotmail.com**

Angelic-Reiki Energy Healing Course Work

And Permission Forms

Copyright © 2019

ISBN 978-1466289215

Where Angels Gather, The Fellowship Inc.

Written By

Rev. Debbie Michaels

All Rights Reserved

No part of this book may be used or reproduced in any manner, including Internet usage, without prior written permission from the author/copyright holder, except in critical articles and reviews

**Contact the author at…**
**AngelsGather88@hotmail.com**

# Course Work Level 1

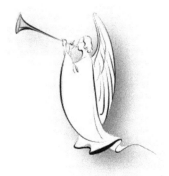

# Chakra System

# Student Course Chakra System

## Angelic Chakra Alignment vs. Standard Chakra Alignment:
What are the difference between Angelic Chakra Alignment and Standard Chakra System?

**Know each color of the Chakras and where they are located:**

**Base/Root:**
Location: _____
Color: _____


**The Sacral:**

Location: _____
Color: _____


**The Solar Plexus:**
Location: _____
Color: _____


**The Heart:**
Location: _____
Color: _____


**TheThroat:**
Location: _____
Color: _____


**The Third Eye/Brow:**
Location: _____
Color: _____


**The Crown:**
Location: _____
Color: _____

**How do you balance your own energy?**

_____
_____
_____
_____
_____
_____
_____
_____
_____
_____
_____
_____
_____
_____
_____
_____
_____
_____
_____
_____
_____
_____
_____
_____
_____
_____
_____
_____

## **Balancing of Standard Chakras**

**Student will perform two A-REH Standard Chakra Balancing:**

Name:_____

Date:_____

Name:_____

Date:_____

# Standard Chakra Chart

| Chakra | Color | Focus Point |
| --- | --- | --- |
| **1 Root Chakra**<br>Located at the base of the spine | Red | Stability, grounding, security, physical energy, will |
| **2 Sacral Chakra**<br>Located below the navel | Orange | Creativity, sexuality reproduction, and desire, emotion |
| **3 Solar Plexus Chakra**<br>Located at solar plexus | Yellow | Intellect, ambition, personal power |
| **4 Heart Chakra**<br>Located at center of the chest | Green | Love, compassion, emotional balance |
| **5 Throat Chakra**<br>Located at the neck | Blue | Communication, expression, divine guidance |
| **6 Third Eye Chakra**<br>Located center of forehead | Indigo | Spiritual awareness, intuition |
| **7 Crown Chakra**<br>Located at the top of the head | Violet | Enlightenment, cosmic consciousness, energy, perfection |

# Aura System

# Student Course Work Aura and Aura Clearing

**What is an Aura?**

**What are the Seven Layers in an Aura and what Chakra are they related to?**

# What do the Colors of the Auras mean?

**Black:** _____
_____

**Green:** _____
_____

**Orange:** _____
_____

**Brown:** _____
_____

**Red:** _____
_____

**Blue:** _____
_____

**Indigo:** _____
_____

**Violet:** _____
_____

**Gold:** _____
_____


# Student will perform two A-REH Aura Scans:

**Name:**_____
**Date:**_____


**Name:**_____
**Date:**_____

## What is the difference between Clearing an Aura and Balancing a Chakra?

_____

## Student will perform two A-REH Auras Clearings:

**Name:**_____
**Date:**_____


**Name:**_____
**Date:**_____

# Angelic-Reiki Aura Color

## Aura Interpretations

There are **6 facets** to perceiving and interpreting the layered energy of an aura. Layers are determined by **color, variations, the shapes, consistencies, clarity and the vibration.**

Most methods of aura reading define particular meanings for each color in the spectrum. For Angelic-Reiki Energy Healing, the list below is used for reading and scanning the aura.

- **BLACK:** Often seen around abused children, divorces, drug addicts and torture victims.

- **GREEN:** Friendly people

- **ORANGE:** Strong motivation

- **YELLOW:** Inspiration

- **BROWN:** Indicates a person with common sense

- **RED:** Short tempered

- **BLUE:** People with this color tend to move slow, but safe and sure

- **INDIGO:** Strong psychic ability

- **VIOLET:** Once again humble people

- **GOLD:** A higher level of consciousness

# Soul Cords and Events Cords

# Student Course Work Soul Cords vs. Event-Cords

**What is the difference between Soul Cords and Event Cords?**

**What is the difference between Spiritual Ties and Spiritual Ribbons?**

_____
_____
_____
_____
_____
_____
_____
_____
_____
_____
_____
_____
_____
_____
_____
_____
_____
_____
_____
_____
_____
_____
_____
_____
_____
_____
_____
_____
_____
_____
_____
_____
_____

**Student will perform two A-REH Soul Cords Releases:**

**Name:**_____
**Date:**_____


**Name:**_____
**Date:**_____

# Angelic-Reiki Energy Healing™
# Soul and Event Cord Release Instructions

We work with the Angelic-Reiki Healing Angels. Begin by calling on The Archangel Raphael; now ask for the Angels of Angelic-Reiki to join you, to become one with you; that you both may become one.

## Prayer for Spiritual Protection

*Guardian Angels of the Heavenly Realm,*
*Circle round protection bound*
*Stand tall guarding our gates*
*Ever keeping safe our fate*
*In all Realms in all Space*
*In all Times*
*Sealed*
*With Grace*

Cover yourself and your client with Angelic-Reiki White Light. You may want to light a white candle at this time to represent this angelic protective energy.

Have your client sit comfortably on a chair facing in the North direction. Spray 3 times above the clients Crown Chakra with Angelic-Reiki Charged Holy Water™ Have the client say the Prayer of Purification.

## Prayer of Purification

*Oh Heavenly Angels*
*Of the Angelic-Reiki Healing Realm*
*Hear this Prayer of Purification*
*Make Ready My Soul*
*Sanctify My Soul*
*That I May Be Made Worthy*
*For Your Gift Of*
*Angelic-Reiki Healing Energy*
*May I Become a Pure Vessel*
*Of Your Most*
*Sacred Healing Energy*
*Grant Favor Upon My Soul*
*Grant Favor Upon Me*

The practitioner then reads the Angelic-Reiki Prayer of Healing

# Angelic-Reiki Prayer of Healing

*I call upon the*
*Angelic-Reiki Healing Angels*
*Let your Divine Healing Energy*
*Enter Me,*
*Pulsate Through Me*
*To cleanse and Balance*
*The Soul*
*Of*
*This*
*Most Sacred Being*

1. Both you and your client should hold the intention that all Soul-Cords and Event-Cords will be released and replaced with positive Angelic-Reiki Energy and ask that these cords be released with harm to none.

2. Then release any Soul-Cords and Event-Cords that the client has sent out, ask that they be returned and replaced with Angelic Energy.

3. The practitioner hands should be approximately six inches away from the client's body and will start by placing their hands over the client, starting at their Crown Chakra.

4. Both the practitioner and the client should visualize the cord gently being released as the practitioner slowly glides their hands down the outline of the client's torso.

5. The practitioner should pass their hand one in the front of the client, and the other at the back, slowly moving them down the client's torso, once they reach the Root/Base Chakra the practitioner should fan their hand outward away for the client and shake the energy of the cords off.

6. The practitioner should now return to the Crown Chakra and glide their hands slowly down the sides of the client, once more when reaching the Root/Base Chakra, fan their hands out and shake the energy off.

7. Some clients who are involved in a negative relationship may feel a popping off of these cords. This will cause the client to view their relationship in the correct light, and change the relationship, by changing themselves; suddenly they will have a completely different outlook on the relationship.

8. Also during the releasing of these cords any and all cords from past lives will be released, along with the Karma that accompanied them.

9. You may have to repeat this procedure a couple of times to make sure you get all of the soul and event cords.

**Remember:** at the end of the healing sessions to use **Angelic-Reiki Energy Healing, Charged Holy Water™**, this **seals the healing process**. **3 spritzes** one spritz at the **Crown Chakra**, the second should be spritzed **over the trunk** of the client, and the third spritz should be at **the foot** of the client.

When completed please offer your client some water to drink, it will help ground them. They may need to sit for a while; this is a good time to offer some spiritual counseling.

**Releasing Soul-Cords and Event-Cords is vital for the Human Being's healing and spiritual growth.**

<u>**Also recommend:**</u> for the client to continue the uses of **Angelic-Reiki Energy Healing, Charged Holy Water™,** for **9 days** after the initial Healing Procedure. This enhances the gentleness of the healing process.

<u>**Remember:**</u> the practitioner should have a small basin of water placed in their Healing Room and a clean hand towel. In the basin should be warm water and a table spoon of Angelic-Reiki Energy Healing, Blessed Energy Balancing Salts™ mixed in it.

**After each Angelic-Reiki Energy Healing, Procedure the practitioner should rinse and dry their hand to neutralize the energy that they have used during the healing session.**

# Meditation

# Meditation:
**Student is required to write a short Healing Meditation.**

# Angelic-Reiki Healing Angels
# Healing Meditation

Remember: You can work with the **Angelic-Reiki Healing Angels and Archangel Raphael** using meditation.

**This Meditation may be used for your personal healing and also for your Clients.**

To prepare Invoke the **Angelic-Reiki Healing Angels and Archangel Raphael**, to please help you open to their **Healing Energy** and support you through the healing process.

Sit comfortably where you will not be disturbed. Begin by grounding and centering yourself. Close your eyes and imagining roots growing from your feet into the Earth.

Follow this simple breathing exercise to relax your physical body: breathe in through your nose, hold it for several seconds, and release it very slowly through your mouth.

Continue breathing this way throughout the meditation.

Ask **The Divine Creator** to send down a beam of protective white light. Envision a beam of light coming down from the Heavens. Watch it surround you and your client, placing you both in a protective sphere.

**This Sphere of White Light is protecting you and your client in all time, all realms, and all space.**

# Course Work Level 2

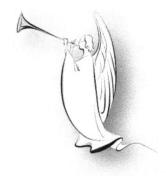

# Divine Energy Flow:

**What is Divine Energy Flow?**

_____
_____
_____
_____
_____
_____
_____
_____
_____
_____
_____
_____
_____
_____
_____
_____

**What are the 12 Meridians and their functions?**

1. **Location and Function:**

    _____
    _____
    _____
    _____
    _____

2. **Location and Function:**

    _____
    _____
    _____
    _____
    _____

3. **Location and Function:**

    _____
    _____
    _____
    _____
    _____

4. **Location and Function:**

    _____
    _____
    _____
    _____
    _____

5. **Location and Function:**

6. **Location and Function:**

7. **Location and Function:**

8. **Location and Function:**

9. **Location and Function:**

10. **Location and Function:**

11. **Location and Function:**

12. **Location and Function:**

# The 12 Meridians

### The Heart Meridian
**The Heart Meridian**, this represents compassion and thus governs emotions and the spirit. It is also responsible for the circulation of the blood and the total body through the brain and the five senses. This meridian is also the mechanism that adapts external stimulation to the body's internal environment.

### The Liver Meridian
**The Liver Meridian**, this meridian stores nutrients and energy for physical activities. It also helps resists against dis-ease and supplies, analyses and detoxifies blood in order to maintain physical energy.

### The Intestine Meridian
**The Intestine Meridian**, this meridian helps the function of the lung, and secretes and excretes from inside and outside the body. It also eliminates the stagnation of energy.

### The Triple Warmer Meridian
The Triple Burner Meridian, this is different from the other meridians because it is not represented by a physical organ. Its purpose is to circulate a water-type energy throughout the other organs. Blockage in the Triple Burner Meridian often manifests itself as a stiff neck or water retention.

**1. The Lung Meridian** – is the intake of Qi energy from the air for use by the body, and to build up resistance against any external intrusions. It also eliminates gasses that are not needed in the body through exhalation.

**3. The Spleen Meridian** – is involved in digestion and the process of fermentation. In modern terms, the spleen is considered as being the pancreas, and the pancreas governs general digestion, and reproductive hormones related to the breasts and ovaries. Mental fatigue has a negative effect on the spleen and a lack of exercise will cause problems with digestion and also with the secretion of hormones.

**4. The Stomach Meridian** – this meridian is involved in the functioning of the stomach, esophagus, and duodenum, as well as the functioning of the reproductive, lactation, ovary, and appetite mechanism. It is also involved in the menstrual cycle.

**6. The Small Intestine Meridian** – the small intestine governs the total body through the displacement and digestion of food. Anxiety, anger, nervous shock, and emotional excitement can affect the circulation of the blood, and the small intestine can actually cause blood stagnation that affects the body as a whole.

**7. The Kidney Meridian** - this meridian controls the spirit and energy to the body and governs resistance against mental stress by controlling hormone secretions. It also detoxifies and purifies the blood.

**8. The Bladder Meridian** – this is related to the mid-brain which cooperates with the kidney system and the pituitary gland. It is also connected to the autonomic nervous system related to the reproductive and urinary organs. It is also responsible for expelling urine.

**9. The Heart Constrictor (Pericardium) Meridian** – this meridian acts as a supplemental function of the heart related to the circulatory system, which includes the heart sac, the cardiac arteries and the system of arteries and veins. It is also responsible for total nutrition.

**12. The Gall Bladder Meridian** – this meridian distributes nutrients throughout the body and balances the total energy through the help of internal hormones and secretions include bile, saliva, gastric acid, insulin, and intestinal hormones.

# Sacred Symbols:

**What is the purpose of Sacred Symbols?**

_____
_____
_____
_____
_____
_____
_____

**What is the function of the 4 Sacred Symbols and who are the Angels connected to them?**

**Body Symbol:**

_____
_____
_____
_____
_____
_____
_____

**Mind Symbol:**

_____
_____
_____
_____
_____
_____
_____

**Emotion Symbol:**

_____
_____
_____
_____
_____
_____
_____

**Soul Symbol:**

_____
_____
_____
_____
_____
_____
_____

**What is the purpose for using A-REH Charged Holy Water?**
_____
_____
_____
_____

**What are the three common steps in performing A-REH™ Energy Healing?**

Step1_____
_____
_____
_____
_____
_____
_____
_____
_____

Step2:_____
_____
_____
_____
_____
_____
_____
_____
_____
_____
_____

Step3:_____
_____
_____
_____
_____
_____
_____
_____
_____
_____
_____

**<u>Performing A-REH™ Energy Healing Secessions:</u>**
Student will perform two A-REH™ Energy Healing Secessions:

**Name:**_____
**Date:**_____


**Name:**_____
**Date:**_____
**<u>Different Variations of A-REH™ Energy Healing:</u>**

**What is Positive Thinking Reinforcement?**

_____
_____
_____
_____
_____
_____
_____
_____
_____
_____
_____
_____
_____
_____
_____
_____
_____
_____
_____

**Explain what the term "Past Life" means and how A-REH™ Energy Healing can help heal the trauma for Past Lives?**

_____
_____
_____
_____
_____
_____
_____
_____
_____
_____
_____
_____
_____
_____
_____
_____

## **Performing A-REH™ Past Lives Secessions:**
**Student will perform two A-REH™ Past Lives Healing Secessions:**

**Name:**_____
**Date:**_____


**Name:**_____
**Date:**_____

**What is A-RDSH and what are the principles of directing A-REH™ Energy?**

_____

## Performing A-RDSH™ Secessions:
Student will perform two A-RDSH™ Secessions:

Name:_____
Date:_____


Name:_____
Date:_____

# 4 Sacred Symbols:

The Sacred Symbols may be drawn over the client, or visualizes them during their treatment. You may also choose to place the **Angelic-Reiki Symbol Cards** in plain view while you are doing a healing session; this will help the practitioner focus.

Another option is for the practitioner to have their client hold a card with the **Angelic-Reiki Energy Healing Symbol** pictured on them; this method is extremely powerful for both the practitioner and their client.

# Body:

**The Angelic-Reiki Energy Healing Symbol "Body"** carries the energy of Angelic-Reiki Realm and Human Being coming together. The primary use of this Sacred Angelic-Reiki Symbol is to increase the healing power for the physical body. It draws the Angelic-Reiki Energies and focuses it to where the healing is required. It can be used for anything, anywhere.

* For on the spot treatments.
* To cleanse negative energies.
* Spiritual protection.
* To aid any physical healing be it structural or biological.
* In sick rooms and hospitals.

**Invoke: Archangel Raphael**

> Envision this sign over the client (or yourself) and say (silently) the words…

**"I ask for Divine Angelic-Reiki Healing Energy to enter this Physical Body of this Sacred Human Being, this most Holy Vessel."**

# Emotions:

**The Angelic-Reiki Energy Healing Symbol "Emotion "** carries the energy of Divine healing power of Love. It is used primarily for emotional healing. It is the Angelic-Reiki Symbol to use for healing the emotions; it empowers the practitioner with Divine Energy of affection, love, compassion, and sympathy. It is used to heal not only a person's emotions but also for the circumstances that the person may be experiencing.

* For on the spot treatments.
* To cleanse negative energies.
* For healing past traumas
* Clears emotional blockages

**Invoke: Archangel Muriel**

> Envision this sign over the client (or yourself) and say (silently) the words…

***"As I am one with Angelic-Reiki Healing Energy, I am secure and at peace with myself, I am whole and complete".***

# Mind:

**The Angelic-Reiki Symbol "Mind** "carries the energy of Divine healing power of Clarity. It is used primarily for mental/emotional healing and calming the mind. It is used for:

* Psychic protection

* Cleansing

* To balance the right and left brain

* Aid for removing addictions

* For healing past traumas

* Removing negative energies and bad vibrations

**Invoke: Archangel Uriel**

> Envision this sign over the client (or yourself) and say (silently) the words…

***"I ask for Clarity, Knowledge, and Wisdom to become one with this Sacred Human Being"***

# Soul:

**The Angelic-Reiki Symbol "Soul"** carries the energy used to heal the soul. Since it deals with the soul and the Human Being's Spiritual Self, it heals dis-ease and illness from the original source. It helps to provide enlightenment and peace. With the use of this Sacred Symbol the Human Being becomes more intuitive and psychic.

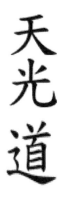

- With repeated use of this most Sacred Symbol you will experience profound life changes.
- Heals the Sacred Human Soul
- Balances the Standard Chakras
- Removes negative energy from all layers of the Aura

**Invoke: Archangel Metatron**

> Envision this sign over the client (or yourself) and say (silently) the words...

*"I accept this Angelic-Reiki Energy Healing. As I am one with The Angelic-Reiki Energy, it Flows freely and in Abundance; Healing the Spirit of this your Most Sacred Human Being."*

# The Fifth Most Sacred:

The Fifth Most Sacred of All Angelic-Reiki Symbol is the **Ordained Master Symbol**. This Most Sacred Symbol is the *central essence of Angelic-Reiki Energy Healing.* **The Fifth Scared Ordained Master Symbol carries the Angelic-Reiki Light of the Ordained Master.**

This Sacred Symbol is given at the Final Attunement; this is part of the Divine Blessing and Infusion of Angelic-Reiki Energy, and signifies the Activation of Angelic-Reiki Healing Energy into the Practitioner.

This Most Sacred of All Symbols will not be found in any other book. It is kept *Sanctified* by the *Ordained Angelic-Reiki Master*; it becomes a part of their Sacred Being, their Sacred Soul. This Symbol is not to be shown to anyone.

The Most Sacred of All
Angelic-Reiki Energy Healing Symbol
Ordained Master Symbol
This Most Sacred Symbol is the Primary Essence of Angelic-Reiki Healing Energy
it carries The Light of the Practitioner's Third and Final Attunement; The Divine
Blessing and Infusion of Angelic-Reiki Healing Energy. It signifies Its' Activation
This Most Sacred of All Symbol will not be found in any book. It is to be kept
Sanctified by the
Ordained Angelic-Reiki Energy Healing Master
This Sacred Symbol becomes a part of
Your
Sacred Being
&
Your Sacred Soul

**Ordained Angelic-Reiki Energy Healing Master
Heaven's Purified Soul with Healing Hands**

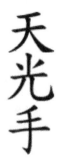

**Congratulations on the competition of your Angelic-Reiki Energy Healing Course.**

**Now begins your calling to humanity and the world.**

**Permission Forms
For Service**

# Release Form for Angelic-Reiki Healing

Practitioner Name_____

Phone Number_____

I understand that Angelic-Reiki is a stress reduction and relaxation energy healing technique. I acknowledge that treatments administered are only for the purpose of helping the client to relax and to release stress. Angelic-Reiki practitioners do not diagnose conditions, nor do they prescribe substances or perform medical treatments, nor interfere with any treatment of a licensed medical professional. It is recommended that I see a licensed physician, or licensed health care professional for any physical or psychological ailment that I may have.

I also understand and believe that the body has the ability to heal itself, and thus, complete relaxation is often beneficial. Long term imbalances in the body sometimes require multiple treatments to allow the body to reach the level of relaxation necessary to bring the systems back into balance. I understand and believe that self-improvement requires commitment on my part, and that I must be willing to change in a positive way if I am to receive the full benefit of any Angelic-Reiki treatment.

**Privacy notice:** No information about any client will be disclosed to any third party without consent of the client and/or parent or guardian of a client who is under the legal age of 18.

**Print Client Name:** _____

**Client Signature:** _____

**Client Phone:** _____

**Client Email:** _____

**Date of Service:** _____

# Client Instructions for Distant Angelic-Reiki Energy Healing

Client should allow at least one hour for Healing Session.

Client should sit or lay quietly when ready to start the Client should recite The Angelic-Reiki Energy Healing Prayer of Purification.

### Prayer of Purification
Oh Heavenly Angels of the Angelic-Reiki Healing Realm
Hear this Prayer of Purification
Make Ready My Soul Sanctify My Soul
That I Man Be Made Worthy for Your Gift of Angelic-Reiki Healing Energy
May I Become a Pure Vessel of Your Most Sacred Healing Energy
Grant Favor upon My Soul Grant Favor upon Me

After the Client recites the Prayer of Purification, he/she should sit or lie quietly and focus on receiving Angelic-Reiki Healing Energy recharging their body. They should start at the by focusing on their toes and slowly moving up the body. At each section of the physical body they should see with their mind's eye the Angelic-Reiki Energy penetrating into their boby.as it is being healed.

Please allow at least 1 hour for this session.

When session is finished please recite "I am thankful for this healing."

The Client should drink some water afterwards at least an 8oz glass, you may feel a little lightheaded for a few minutes, please rest before moving around quickly.

The Client may also want to take a bath or shower afterwards, if you do please place some Sea Salt or Epson Salt in the water to help you balance and ground you.

What the practitioner will be doing…

During the designated time the practitioner will be preforming the Distance Angelic-Reiki Energy Healing. The practitioner will be sending the client Healing Energies of the Angelic-Reiki Healing Angels.

# Release Form for Aura Scanning and Cleansing

Practitioner Name_____

Phone Number_____

I understand that Angelic-Reiki is a stress reduction and relaxation energy healing technique. I acknowledge that treatments administered are only for the purpose of helping the client to relax and to release stress. Aura Scanning and Cleansing is one of the many treatments available with Angelic-Reiki. Angelic-Reiki practitioners do not diagnose conditions, nor do they prescribe substances or perform medical treatments, nor interfere with any treatment of a licensed medical professional. It is recommended that I see a licensed physician, or licensed health care professional for any physical or psychological ailment that I may have.

I also understand and believe that the body has the ability to heal itself, and thus, complete relaxation is often beneficial. Long term imbalances in the body sometimes require multiple treatments to allow the body to reach the level of relaxation necessary to bring the systems back into balance. I understand and believe that self-improvement requires commitment on my part, and that I must be willing to change in a positive way if I am to receive the full benefit of any Angelic-Reiki treatment.

**Privacy notice:** No information about any client will be disclosed to any third party without consent of the client and/or parent or guardian of a client who is under the legal age of 18.

**Print Client Name:** _____

**Client Signature:** _____

**Client Phone:** _____

**Client Email:** _____

**Date of Service:** _____

# Client Instructions for Distant Angelic-Reiki Energy Healing Aura Scan and Clearing

Client should allow at least one hour for Healing Session.

Client should sit or lay quietly when ready to start the Client should recite The Angelic-Reiki Energy Healing Prayer of Purification.

### Prayer of Purification
Oh Heavenly Angels of the Angelic-Reiki Healing Realm
Hear this Prayer of Purification
Make Ready My Soul Sanctify My Soul
That I Man Be Made Worthy for Your Gift of Angelic-Reiki Healing Energy
May I Become a Pure Vessel of Your Most Sacred Healing Energy
Grant Favor upon My Soul Grant Favor Upon Me

After the Client recites the Prayer of Purification, he/she should sit or lie quietly and focus on receiving Angelic-Reiki Healing Energy recharging their Aura. They should start at the by focusing on their inner being and focus the damage energies clearing out and radiating clean healthy energies with all holes in their energy field being healed.

Please allow at least 1 hour for this session.

When session is finished please recite "I am thankful for this healing."

The Client should drink some water afterwards at least an 8oz glass, you may feel a little lightheaded for a few minutes, please rest before moving around quickly.

The Client may also want to take a bath or shower afterwards, if you do please place some Sea Salt or Epson Salt in the water to help you balance and ground you.

What the practitioner will be doing...

During the designated time the practitioner will be preforming the Distance Angelic-Reiki Energy Healing. The practitioner will be sending the client Healing Energies of the Angelic-Reiki Healing Angels.

# Release Form for Balancing Chakras

Practitioner Name_____

Phone Number_____


I understand that Angelic-Reiki is a stress reduction and relaxation energy healing technique. I acknowledge that treatments administered are only for the purpose of helping the client to relax and to release stress. Balancing Chakras is one of the many treatments available with Angelic-Reiki. Angelic-Reiki practitioners do not diagnose conditions, nor do they prescribe substances or perform medical treatments, nor interfere with any treatment of a licensed medical professional. It is recommended that I see a licensed physician, or licensed health care professional for any physical or psychological ailment that I may have.

I also understand and believe that the body has the ability to heal itself, and thus, complete relaxation is often beneficial. Long term imbalances in the body sometimes require multiple treatments to allow the body to reach the level of relaxation necessary to bring the systems back into balance. I understand and believe that self-improvement requires commitment on my part, and that I must be willing to change in a positive way if I am to receive the full benefit of any Angelic-Reiki treatment.

**Privacy notice:** No information about any client will be disclosed to any third party without consent of the client and/or parent or guardian of a client who is under the legal age of 18.


**Print Client Name:** _____

**Client Signature:** _____

**Client Phone:** _____

**Client Email:** _____

**Date of Service:** _____

# Client Instructions for Distant Angelic-Reiki Energy Healing Chakra Balancing

Client should allow at least one hour for Healing Session.

Client should sit or lay quietly when ready to start the Client should recite The Angelic-Reiki Energy Healing Prayer of Purification.

## Prayer of Purification

Oh Heavenly Angels of the Angelic-Reiki Healing Realm
Hear this Prayer of Purification
Make Ready My Soul Sanctify My Soul
That I Man Be Made Worthy for Your Gift of Angelic-Reiki Healing Energy
May I Become a Pure Vessel of Your Most Sacred Healing Energy
Grant Favor upon My Soul Grant Favor Upon Me

After the Client recites the Prayer of Purification, he/she should sit or lie quietly and focus on receiving Angelic-Reiki Healing Energy recharging their Chakra System starting with the Crown Chakra and working down. Please focus on a brilliant violet light penetrating through the top on the head and filling the complete body and soul. Each Chakra should be focused on for at least 10 minutes. Please allow at least 1 and a half hour for this session.

When session is finished please recite "I am thankful for this healing."

The Client should drink some water afterwards at least an 8oz glass, you may feel a little lightheaded for a few minutes, please rest before moving around quickly.

The Client may also want to take a bath or shower afterwards, if you do please place some Sea Salt or Epson Salt in the water to help you balance and ground you.

What the practitioner will be doing…

During the designated time the practitioner will be preforming the Distance Angelic-Reiki Energy Healing. The practitioner will be sending the client Healing Energies of the Angelic-Reiki Healing Angels.

# Release Form for Releasing Soul-Cords and Event-Cords

Practitioner Name_____

Phone Number_____

I understand that Angelic-Reiki is a stress reduction and relaxation energy healing technique. I acknowledge that treatments administered are only for the purpose of helping the client to relax and to release stress. Releasing Soul-Cords and Event-Cords is one of the many treatments available with Angelic-Reiki. Angelic-Reiki practitioners do not diagnose conditions, nor do they prescribe substances or perform medical treatments, nor interfere with any treatment of a licensed medical professional. It is recommended that I see a licensed physician, or licensed health care professional for any physical or psychological ailment that I may have.

I also understand and believe that the body has the ability to heal itself, and thus, complete relaxation is often beneficial. Long term imbalances in the body sometimes require multiple treatments to allow the body to reach the level of relaxation necessary to bring the systems back into balance. I understand and believe that self-improvement requires commitment on my part, and that I must be willing to change in a positive way if I am to receive the full benefit of any Angelic-Reiki treatment.

**Privacy notice:** No information about any client will be disclosed to any third party without consent of the client and/or parent or guardian of a client who is under the legal age of 18.

**Print Client Name:** _____

**Client Signature:** _____

**Client Phone:** _____

**Client Email:** _____

**Date of Service:** _____

# Client Instructions for Distant Angelic-Reiki Energy Healing Soul and Event Cord Release

Client should allow at least one hour for Healing Session.

Client should sit or lay quietly when ready to start the Client should recite The Angelic-Reiki Energy Healing Prayer of Purification.

### Prayer of Purification
Oh Heavenly Angels of the Angelic-Reiki Healing Realm
Hear this Prayer of Purification
Make Ready My Soul Sanctify My Soul
That I Man Be Made Worthy for Your Gift of Angelic-Reiki Healing Energy
May I Become a Pure Vessel of Your Most Sacred Healing Energy
Grant Favor upon My Soul Grant Favor Upon Me

After the Client recites the Prayer of Purification, he/she should sit or lie quietly and focus on releasing all Cords gently.

Please allow at least 1 hour for this session.

When session is finished please recite "I am thankful for this healing."

The Client should drink some water afterwards at least an 8oz glass, you may feel a little lightheaded for a few minutes, please rest before moving around quickly.

The Client may also want to take a bath or shower afterwards, if you do please place some Sea Salt or Epson Salt in the water to help you balance and ground you.

What the practitioner will be doing…

During the designated time the practitioner will be preforming the Distance Angelic-Reiki Energy Healing. The practitioner will be sending the client Healing Energies of the Angelic-Reiki Healing Angels.

# Angelic-Reiki Hand Placement Chart

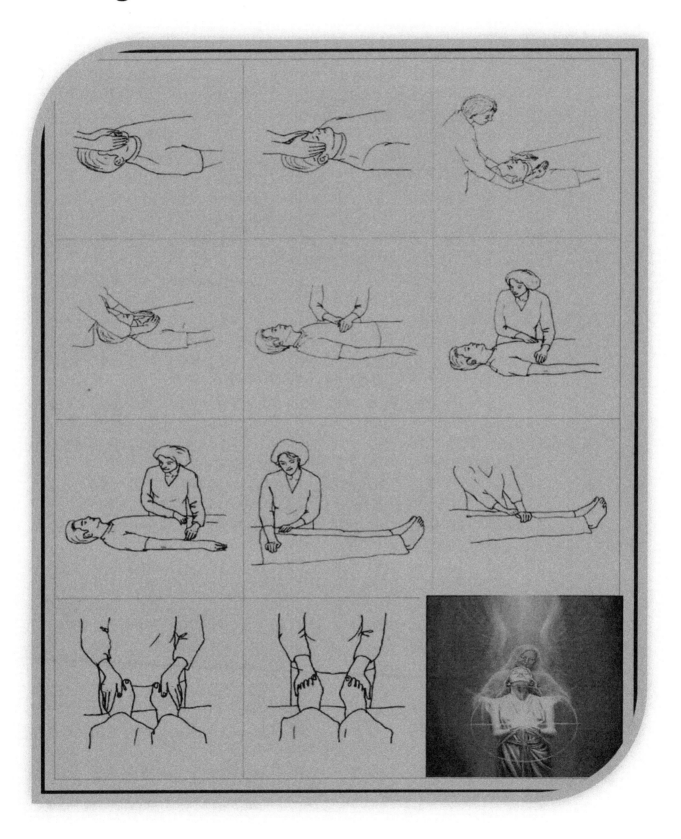

CPSIA information can be obtained
at www.ICGtesting.com
Printed in the USA
LVHW061416111119
636961LV00020B/5481/P